Thyroid Healing

The Proven 4 Week Program to Improve Your Metabolism, Hypothyroidism, Hormones, Tiredness, and Weight Gain

With Amy Room MD

Aviva William PharmD

George Myers MD

THYROID HEALING

Copyright © 2020 George Myers MD

Table of Contents

ACKNOWLEDGMENTS.. 4

INTRODUCTION... 5

PART 1.. 5

CHAPTER 1: WHAT IN THE WORLD IS A THYROID 6

CHAPTER 2: POSSIBLE THYROID DISORDERS 14

    Hyperthyroidism...14

    Hypothyroidism..22

    Hashimoto's Disease..36

    Graves' Disease..40

    Goiter...45

PART 2... 54

CHAPTER 1: WHAT IS THE ALKALINE DIET 55

CHAPTER 2: WHAT IS A PH BALANCE?..................................... 59

CHAPTER 3: THE SCIENCE BEHIND PH IMBALANCE.............. 63

CHAPTER 4: WHY ALKALINE IS BEST....................................... 67

CHAPTER 5: CREATING AN ACID-ALKALINE BALANCE......... 71

CHAPTER 6: ALKALINE DIET FOR VEGETARIANS 75

CHAPTER 7: ALKALINE MEAL IDEAS... 79

CONCLUSION 83

Acknowledgments

We would like to acknowledge the American Thyroid Association and the hard work of everyone involved in the prevention and treatment of any and all thyroid conditions, which affect the health and lives of many loved ones. Thank you.

Introduction

The reasons to pick up a book of this sort are many. Perhaps you have picked this title because you are currently suffering from an issue with your thyroid gland. Maybe you have in the past and wish to get a greater understanding of what it was that you went through. Or you may even just want to be prepared for the eventuality and desire the knowledge necessary to prevent an issue with the thyroid gland of yourself or your loved ones from occurring altogether.

Whatever your reasons, whatever it is you are seeking to gain from choosing this text, it will provide you with the answers and with needed help. For it is easy to overlook or not keep in mind the thyroid gland despite its importance and role in the maintenance of our health.

Conditions afflicting the thyroid gland are in no way scarce and can be made to become quite severe, if and when left unattended to in the proper manner, or by the proper medical authorities. With that in mind do not worry, there is no need to feel intimidated or overly cautious about diving into this subject matter. You have already taken the correct first steps in supplementing and elevating the health of your thyroid gland. You have picked up this title and chosen to become more informed and play a more active role when it comes to the health of your thyroid gland, yourself and your body.

Thank you for doing so, and please enjoy

PART 1

Chapter 1: What in The World Is A Thyroid

In this chapter, we will be exploring just what the thyroid is, and its functions in maintaining and keeping your body healthy.

For starters, the word thyroid has its origins dating as far back as the 1690s. Coming from the Greek, *thyreoiedes*, meaning "shield-shaped". Also referred to as, *khondros thyreoiedes*, "shield-shaped cartilage". Aptly named, as the thyroid gland is an organ which is often considered to resemble a butterfly, bow tie, or shield shape, at the base of the neck.

The thyroid gland plays an extremely vital role in the way your body uses energy, by releasing hormones that aid in controlling your body's metabolism. The hormones released by the thyroid gland assist in regulating important body functions, including but not limited to:

- Regulation of breathing
- Heart rate
- The central and peripheral nervous systems
- Body weight
- Cycles of menstruation
- The strength of muscles
- Levels of cholesterol
- The temperature of the body

Quite a lot for an organ coming in at only around 2 inches long. This tiny but important gland rests in the front portion of the throat, in front of the trachea, and just below the thyroid cartilage commonly referred to as the

Adam's apple. The Adam's apple itself is the largest cartilage of the voice box or larynx.

Owing to the bow tie, butterfly, or shield shape, of the thyroid gland, is a middle connection of thin thyroid tissue, which is known as the isthmus, which is responsible for holding together two lobes on the right and left sides of it. It is not entirely uncommon, however, for someone to be missing the isthmus all-together and instead of having the two lobes of the thyroid gland operating separate from one another.

Now that you are aware of this and may feel a bit more familiar with your own thyroid gland, you may resist trying to see or feel around for it in your neck yourself. Unless the thyroid gland is otherwise afflicted and made to become enlarged, mostly known as a goiter, the thyroid will be unable to be seen, and only just barely able to be felt. It is only when a goiter occurs and the neck is swollen from an enlarged thyroid that it will be at all noticeable either to the eye or to the touch.

The thyroid gland is one of the major players in the endocrine system. The endocrine system includes glands that are responsible for the production and for the secretion of various hormones. The other organs which help make up the endocrine system are the hypothalamus, which is responsible for linking the body's nervous system to the endocrine system via the use of the pituitary gland. The pituitary gland which is responsible for the secretion of hormones, not the blood stream. The pineal gland, which produces the wake/sleep pattern hormone of melatonin. The adrenal glands, which are responsible for the production of a variety of hormones like the steroids cortisol and aldosterone as well as our body's adrenaline.

The Pancreas, an organ located in the abdominal region of the body, the primary role of which is the converting of food into fuel for the body's cells. The ovaries and testicles, sex organs of the body. And the parathyroid glands.

Utilizing the iodine content from foods, the thyroid is able to produce and churn out the hormones T3, which stands for triiodothyronine, and the hormone T4, thyroxine.

T3, or triiodothyronine, is merely the active form of the companion hormone thyroxine, or T4. The thyroid gland alone is able to secrete around 20% of our body's T3 into the bloodstream on its own. With the other 80% coming from organs like the liver and the kidneys going through the process of converting thyroxine into its active counterpart.

It is absolutely possible for your body to have far too much of T3 though. When there is an over secretion of T3 into the blood stream, it is called thyrotoxicosis. This can be due to a number of conditions dealing with the thyroid gland such as overactivity in the thyroid gland, known as hyperthyroidism, caused by such conditions as a benign tumor, the thyroid gland becoming enflamed, or a condition known as graves' disease. The previously mentioned condition of a goiter, in which the neck begins to swell, might be a signal of thyrotoxicosis having occurred. Even more symptoms to have an eye out for in case of hyperthyroidism will be an increase in the appetite, increased regularity of bowel movements, an intolerance to heat, the loss of weight, the menstrual cycle becoming irregulated, a heartbeat becoming increasingly rapid or irregular in rhythm, the thinning or loss of hair, tremors, becoming irritable, overly tired, palpitations, and the eyelids retracting.

It is also possible for your body to be producing too little of the hormone T3. The thyroid gland producing too little of T3 is known commonly as hypothyroidism. It is common for autoimmune diseases to have a strong role in this occurring, an example of which would be the Hashimoto's disease, which causes the immune system to attack the thyroid gland. Certain medications or the intake of too little iodine can also cause hypothyroidism. This can be very serious, especially if a case of hypothyroidism goes unnoticed or untreated during early childhood, or even before birth. With the regulation of hormones being so important, primarily to physical and mental development, not treating hypothyroidism during these crucial times often result in reduced growth for the child, or becoming learning disabled.

The affliction of hypothyroidism is not foreign to adults though. When hypothyroidism occurs in adults they tend to have the functions of their bodies slowed down drastically. The effects of hypothyroidism in an adult have been known to include symptoms such as a growing intolerance to colder temperature, the heart rate of the adult will lower, gaining weight, a reduction in appetite, the ability of memory becomes poorer, fertility will reduce, muscles will become stiff, the adult may become depressed, and tired.

T4, or thyroxine, is the primary hormone that gets secreted from the thyroid gland and into the body's bloodstream. Unlike T3 which is active, thyroxine is in an inactive form and most of it will need to be converted to the active form, triiodothyronine, which is a process that takes place in organs like the kidneys and liver. Undergoing these processes is vital in making sure the body is able to regulate a healthy metabolic rate, control of the body's muscles, development of the brain, develop and maintain bones, and digestive and heart functionality.

As with T3, triiodothyronine, the production and secretion of too much will inevitable result in thyrotoxicosis, while the production and secretion of too little thyroxine, will result in hypothyroidism.

To combat this, the body and thyroid gland have a few tricks vital to the regulation of levels of these hormones in the cells. There is a controlled feedback loop system, involving the hypothalamus in the brain as well as in the thyroid gland and pituitary gland which is in control of the production of both of the hormones thyroxine and triiodothyronine. Thyrotropin-releasing hormones are secreted from the hypothalamus and, in turn, the pituitary gland becomes stimulated into producing thyroid stimulating hormone. A hormone which will stimulate thyroxine and triiodothyronine to be produced and secreted by the thyroid gland.

A feedback loop regulates this production system, to account for the levels of thyroxine and of triiodothyronine. If the levels of either of these thyroid gland hormones begin to increase, they will end up preventing the production and secretion of the thyrotropin-releasing hormone as well as the thyroid stimulating hormone, thus allowing the body to maintain, on it's own, a steady level of the thyroid hormones that it needs.

For all these reasons it is of vital importance that the levels of T3 and T4 being secreted thru-ought the body and its cells never get too high or too low. T3 and T4 are able to reach just about ever cell in the body by utilizing the bloodstream. The rate of work for the cells and metabolism to work is regulated by the hormones T3 and T4. To make sure that levels are never either too high or too low, this is why we have a thyroid gland.

The final hormone that the thyroid gland is responsible for the production of is the hormone calcitonin, CT, or thyrocalcitonin. Within the thyroid gland are what are known as C-cells, or parafollicular cells, which are in charge of the proliferation of this particular hormone. The primary role of calcitonin in the body is to help in the regulation of the levels of phosphate in the blood, and of calcium in the blood. Doing so is to be in opposition of the parathyroid hormone. In short, meaning that what it aims to do is reduce the amount of calcium in the blood stream. The reason for playing this role in the human anatomy game has been a bit of a mystery to science up to this point though, due to the observation of patients showing either very high or even very low levels of the hormone calcitonin, having no adverse effect on them.

The hormone calcitonin has two primary mechanisms by which to aid in the reduction of calcium levels within the human body. It can completely inhibit the activity of the cells in our body which are responsible for breaking down bones, known as osteoclasts. Osteoclasts do this because when bone is broken down, the calcium within the bone being broken down will be released into the body's bloodstream. So by inhibiting the osteoclasts from doing their respective jobs, calcitonin is directly involved in the reduction of the amount of calcium that is getting released into the body's bloodstream. Despite doing this though, the length of time that calcitonin can cause this inhibition has been shown to be quite short.

Calcitonin can be an active player in the resorption of calcium into the kidneys, which it does by lower the levels of blood calcium in the body.

Calcitonin has been manufactured in the past and has then been given, in this form, to treat the disease of bone, Paget's disease. Also known as osteitis deformans, Paget's disease is rather common, and is a chronic bone disorder which can cause pain, fractures or deformities of a bone, or show absolutely no symptoms at all. It is however easily able to be controlled and treated with proper early enough diagnosis and treatment.

The manufactured hormone calcitonin has also been given to sufferers of general bone pain, and of hypercalcaemia, which is when the body has an abnormal level of calcium flowing in the bloodstream.

Though because of the introduction of bisphosphonates, which aid in the preventing of the breakdown of bone cells and are drugs also used to help treat osteoporosis, the use of manufactured calcitonin has decreased.

Chapter 2: Possible Thyroid Disorders

In the previous chapter, we began to cover what it is exactly that the thyroid gland gets done and even dabbled a bit into how it does it's job properly. During the last chapter, we mentioned a few of the various thigs which can afflict the thyroid gland, why this may occur in certain circumstances, and what the effects of these afflictions could be. Moving on into chapter two is where we will begin to take a closer look at everything that can go wrong with the thyroid gland. Not just the what, but the why as well. What causes these changes in our thyroid gland to occur, and what to expect to happen when they do occur. The importance of having this knowledge be a part of your thyroid gland arsenal cannot be at all overstated as there is a wide array of severity to both the symptoms and to the results of the ailments that can afflict the thyroid gland and consequently hinder our body's ability to maintain its health properly.

Just as well in this chapter, you can expect to be reading deeper into some of the ailments that may have already been brought up in the previous chapter, such as hyperthyroidism, hypothyroidism, graves disease, goiters, and Hashimoto's disease.

Hyperthyroidism

As briefly discussed in the last chapter, hyperthyroidism is a rather common condition in which there is overactivity in the thyroid gland and begins to produce far too much of the thyroid hormone which would usually be used to regulate the body's metabolic rate. This can be an overproduction of the hormones T3, which is triiodothyronine, T4, which is tetraiodothyronine, or even an overproduction of both of these hormones.

The causes of hyperthyroidism can vary greatly, with the most common reason for it being the aforementioned Grave's disease, which we will go much further into later in the chapter. The basics of Grave's disease are that it is an autoimmune disorder which causes antibodies in the body to stimulate the thyroid gland making it secrete to many of it's hormones. You should tell your regular doctor if any one in your family has ever had Grave's disease as it seems to have a genetic link, being passed down commonly from generation to the next generation. Grave's disease is also known to be more prevalent in women, affecting about 1 percent of the female population, than it is in men.

Another common reason for hyperthyroidism to occur is an excess level of iodine in the body, which is the main ingredient in hormones T3 and T4.

Less common, but still just as relevant to the conversation as causes for hyperthyroidism is thyroiditis which is the inflammation of thyroid gland, which in turn will cause the hormones T3 and T4 to start leaking out of the thyroid gland.

Tumors located on the ovaries or testes have been known links to hyperthyroidism. As well as even tumors, even when benign, located on the thyroid gland, or pituitary gland.

An easily preventable cause of hyperthyroidism which should not be overlooked is the intake of large amounts of T4, or tetraiodothyronine, via the ingestion of a dietary supplement or of a prescribed medication.

When it comes to the symptoms of hyperthyroidism, believe it or not, we had only scratched the surface in the previous chapter and will be going more in-depth here on what you can expect to look out for in order to self-diagnose an issue before going to seek out a professional opinion.

To begin with, in the case of Grave's disease, one of the symptoms can be a bulging of the eyes as if stuck in a stare. Other symptoms to watch out for would be an increase in the appetite, perhaps an increase in nervousness or a sense of restlessness. Muscular weakness, the inability to concentrate on simple tasks, irregularity in the heartbeat, loss of the ability to sleep soundly or for long periods of time, the loss of hair, or noticing that your hair has become thinner or more brittle, can be signs of hyperthyroidism. Thinness of the skin is also common, as well as becoming more irritable, sweating more, or becoming more anxious. In men specifically, the development of breasts can be a sign of hyperthyroidism. And in women, hyperthyroidism has been known to have adverse effects on the regularity of the menstrual cycle.

If you experience any of the prior symptoms, it is, of course, recommended to seek out professional help and diagnosis. However, it is highly recommended that you seek out professional help for the treatment of hyperthyroidism if you begin to experience a sensation of dizziness if you start to notice shortness in your breathing, which will likely come with the increase in heart rate, making it faster and irregular, and any loss of consciousness. Having hyperthyroidism has also been known to be the cause of atrial fibrillations, which are a dangerous arrythmia, commonly responsible for leading to having a stroke, or even to congestive heart failures.

In diagnosing a case of hyperthyroidism, a doctor will likely begin the process by conducting a full and complete medical history, as well as a physical exam. These are commonly conducted as they are helpful in revealing the common signs of loss of weight, how rapid your pulse is, an elevation in pressure of the blood, protrusion of the eyes, or the enlargement of the thyroid gland itself.

It is also reasonable to expect your doctor to conduct a cholesterol test which will be done to check on the levels of cholesterol in your system. This is done because cholesterol levels being low can be an indication that there is an elevation in your metabolic rate, which would mean that your body is burning through your cholesterol far too quickly.

Doctors are also able to conduct tests to measure the levels of T3 and T4 that are in your blood. Thyroid stimulating hormone tests can be done to check the levels of TSH, or thyroid stimulating hormone coursing within your body. TSH stimulates your thyroid gland to produce the hormones the body needs, and if your thyroid gland is producing levels of hormones at a normal rate, or even a rate that is too high, your TSH should come out lower. And a level of TSH that is abnormally low can be an important signifier that you may have hyperthyroidism.

A triglyceride test will be done, because similarly to having low amounts of cholesterol, a low level of triglycerides can be significant of an elevation in your metabolic rate. A thyroid scan or uptake will allow a doctor to see if your thyroid gland is being overactive. It will actually get even more particular, and let a doctor be able to see if it is the entire thyroid gland which is acting up or just a particular area of the thyroid gland.

Ultrasounds have been known to be utilized, as they will allow a doctor to observe entirely, the size of the thyroid gland, as well as any masses that may be within the thyroid gland. It is the use of the ultrasound which will also be able to let the doctor know if the mass inside the thyroid gland is cystic, or if it is solid. Just as well a CT, Computed Tomography, or MRI, Magnetic Resonance Imaging, scan can be performed to show if the condition is being caused by a tumor being present on the pituitary gland.

Treatment of hyperthyroidism also comes in varieties and may be dependent on the cause of the hyperthyroidism. Perhaps the most common treatment comes in the form of medication. Generally an antithyroid medication like methimazole, also known as Tapazole, which will cause the thyroid gland to halt the production and secretion of hormones altogether.

According to the American Thyroid Association, around 70 percent of U.S. adults who undergo treatment for hyperthyroidism will receive a form of treatment called radioactive iodine. Radioactive iodine is essentially able to completely and effectively destroy the cells that would otherwise be producing hormones. Radioactive iodine, or RAI, in the form of a liquid or a pill, will be ingested by way of the mouth, and is safe to use on an individual who has had any allergic reaction to an X-ray contrast agent or to seafood, because essentially the reaction comes from the compound which contains iodine, and not from the iodine itself. The iodine, in an iodide form, is actually split into two forms or radioactive iodine, known as I-123, which is harmless to thyroid gland cells, and I-131, which is responsible for the destruction of thyroid gland cells. The radiation which is emitted by both of these forms of the iodine are able to be detected from outside of the patient, which will help the doctor to gain any information needed the thyroid glands functionality, and take any pictures needed of the size thyroid glands tissues, as well as their location in the body. This treatment is not without its side effects though, which generally tend to come in the presence of dryness of the mouth, soreness of the eyes and in the throat, and has also been known to effect changes in taste. You may also be required, if undergoing this treatment, to take precautions for a short time which will prevent the spread of radiation to others.

Surgery is yet another common form of treatment for hyperthyroidism. In this case, it is entirely possible that a section of your thyroid gland will be removed, though entire thyroid glands have also been removed in this procedure. This is followed up with taking thyroid hormone supplements which will help in the prevention of hypothyroidism, which is what happens when there is the occurrence of underactivity in the thyroid gland, causing it to produce and secrete too little of the intended hormones. Beta-blockers may also be taken, such as something like propranolol to help control a rapid pulse, sweating, any anxiety that may crop up, and higher blood pressure. It is reported that most people respond very well to this form of treatment.

If you would like to improve any symptoms, or even take action to prevent symptoms from occurring, you are not left without options. You can work along with your doctor, or a dietician, to help create a healthy guideline for diet, exercise, and any nutritional supplementation. Proper diet intake, with a stronger focus on getting calcium and sodium, can be crucially important in the prevention of hyperthyroidism. Osteoporosis is a common result of hyperthyroidism as it can make your bones become thin, weak, and very brittle. To strengthen the bones after treatment for hyperthyroidism, it is recommended to take calcium supplements and vitamin D. To get an idea of how much vitamin D you should be taking post-surgery, you can talk to your doctor for a recommendation.

Moving on from treatment, it is not unusual for a doctor to recommend their patients to an endocrinologist, who will be more specialized in the treatment of systems dealing with bodily hormones. You'll want to avoid stress at this stage as it can cause thyroid storm, which happens when a large amount of thyroid hormone gets released, resulting in a horrible and sudden worsening of any prior symptoms. Proper treatment is both recommended and effective at the prevention of thyroid storm, as well as other complications such as thyrotoxicosis.

In the long-term, the outlook for something like hyperthyroidism is dependent heavily on what is causing it. Some of the causes of hyperthyroidism can go away without ever seeking treatment. Whereas a more serious cause like Graves' disease is not to be taken lightly, as it will get much worse if it goes without treatment, and the complications due to Graves' disease are often life-threatening and will have an affect on your quality of life long-term. These are easy enough to subdue with proper care and an early diagnosis and treatment.

THYROID HEALING

Hypothyroidism

Though we went over a little about hypothyroidism in chapter 1, it is important to take a closer look at the disorder, to gain a better idea of its symptoms, and proper treatment and care for it.

When the body is not producing enough of the thyroid hormones that it needs, this is what is known as hypothyroidism having occurred. This will cause the general functions of your body to become slowed down, as the thyroid gland is responsible for producing and secreting hormones which will provide energy to nearly every other portion of your body. Though this affliction can come to task at any age, it is more common for an underactive thyroid gland to be noticed in adults over the age of 60, as well as being more prevalent in women. A diagnosis of hypothyroidism is nothing to get too worked up about, fortunately, as treatment of hypothyroidism has been known to be quite effective, as well as being very simple and very safe.

Though the symptoms of having an underactive thyroid gland can vary from person to person, there is enough overlap in the symptoms for us to help lay out what to look out for. It is important to note, however, that there can be difficulty in pin-pointing that a symptom is that of hypothyroidism and that the severity of the condition itself plays a large role in which signs or symptoms will appear, as well as when they may make an appearance.

It is not at all uncommon for most people to experience the symptoms of this condition arriving in a slow progression over many years. The thyroid gland will grow ever slower and slower, which will only then allow the symptoms to be better identifiable. The trouble can become that many of the symptoms come with general aging, so if you suspect there is more to the picture, and that hypothyroidism is at play, it is important to go see a doctor. An example of some early symptoms which also come naturally with age are the symptomatic fatigue and gaining of weight.

If hypothyroidism does occur, however, other symptoms to keep an eye out for will be an uptick in depression, constipation, or muscle weakness. It is also common to begin becoming more sensitive to the cold, for the skin to become dry, and a reduction in sweating. Your heart rate will generally become slower, blood cholesterol may elevate, and joints may become stiff or experience more pain. It is also possible for memory to start becoming impaired, hair may thin or become dry. Your voice may become hoarse, muscles will stiffen and experience soreness, your face will become puffy and sensitive. In women, hypothyroidism as been known to negatively affect menstrual changes and cause difficulty in fertility.

When it comes to the causes of hypothyroidism, an autoimmune disease is fairly common to be the culprit at work. The body is designed in such a way that your immune system generally will protect the body's cells against any invading bacteria and virus. Therefore, when an unknown virus or bacteria enters the body, it is the immune system which will respond by sending out what are known as fighter cells, to destroy the foreign invading virus or bacteria.

However, it is not impossible for your body to begin confusing what are the healthy and normal cells, with the invading cells. This is what is then called an autoimmune response to the cells. And if this autoimmune response does not get properly treated, or if it is not properly regulated, it is your own immune system which will start to attack your healthy body tissues. Medically, this has been known to cause quite serious issues, which include hypothyroidism.

Hashimoto's disease, which we have mentioned before, is one such autoimmune condition that can occur, and it is the most common among the causes of having an underactive thyroid gland. The disease literally will attack the thyroid gland which will cause chronic thyroid inflammation, which, in turn, will reduce the functionality of the thyroid gland. As with Graves' disorder having links between generations, it is not at all uncommon to find that multiple members of a family have this same condition as well.

Hypothyroidism can even become an occurrence as a result of treatment for hyperthyroidism, which has the aim of lowering your thyroid hormone. It is not uncommon for the treatment to result in keeping the thyroid hormone too low, which then becomes hypothyroidism, which has been a known result of the radioactive iodine treatment for hyperthyroidism.

The surgical removal of the thyroid gland is yet another known cause of the occurrence of hypothyroidism. The entirety of the thyroid gland will be removed in the case of thyroid problems cropping up, which will affect the body's ability to produce thyroid hormone, and cause hypothyroidism. In this instance, you will typically be recommended to take thyroid medication for the rest of your life. In the case that it is only a smaller portion of the thyroid gland which is removed, it is possible for the thyroid gland to still be able to produce and secrete a healthy amount of hormones. In which case it will take a test of the blood to determine how much medication you will need.

It is possible for radiation therapy to be the cause if you have come down with hypothyroidism. A diagnosis of leukemia, neck cancer, or lymphoma will likely mean you have had to undergo a form of radiation therapy, which very nearly almost leads to the occurrence of hypothyroidism.

Just as possible, is a medication you may be taking to lower thyroid gland hormone production, to be the cause of hypothyroidism. Medications such as these are commonly used in the treatment of certain psychological diseases, and even have been known to be used in treating heart disease and cancer.

When it comes down the diagnosing of hypothyroidism, there are two primary methods which have been favored and work to best identify when it has occurred. The first being a strict medical evaluation, much like in the case of checking for hyperthyroidism. The doctor will give you a very thorough exam physically, as well as making sure to go over your medical history. Hypothyroidism has a couple physical signs which the doctor will be checking for primarily such as the dryness of the skin, how slow or quick your reflexes are, any swelling of the neck, and the rate of your heart beat. It is at this time that a doctor will also likely ask you to report any of the other symptoms listed earlier that you may have experienced, such as the depression, any fatigue, if you have been constipated, and a sensation of being more sensitive to the cold. It is also at this point it will be most helpful for you to let the doctor know of any thyroid conditions which have existed in your family.

To reliably get an idea of the existence of hypothyroidism in the body, it is required to conduct blood tests. It is only by this method that anyone will be able to tell and get a look at a measure of your body's thyroid-stimulating hormone levels, done by utilizing a thyroid-stimulating hormone test to see how much of the thyroid-stimulating hormone your pituitary gland is or is not creating. In the case that your thyroid gland is not producing enough of the hormone, the pituitary gland will respond to this by boosting the thyroid-stimulating hormone it produces in order to increase thyroid hormone production. If it turns out you have hypothyroidism, the levels of thyroid-stimulating hormone in your body will be increased, because your body is responding by making an attempt at stimulating more thyroid gland hormone activity. If hyperthyroidism is what ails you, the levels of the thyroid-stimulating hormone in your body will as having decreased, because in this case, your body has begun the process of attempting to halt the function of excessive production of the thyroid glands hormones.

Another useful method in the detection and diagnosis of hypothyroidism is to test the levels of T4 in the body, being produced by your thyroid gland, as T4 is produced directly by the thyroid gland. When they are used in conjunction with one another, a test of T4 levels and the thyroid-stimulating hormone test are very helpful in coming up with an evaluation of thyroid gland functionality. In general, if you the levels of thyroid-stimulating hormone in your body has increased, while the level of the hormone T4 has decreased, you much more than likely have hypothyroidism. Though, due to the sheer amount of conditions that can have such a negative impact on the thyroid gland, it could very well end up being necessary to conduct even more tests of the thyroid glands function I order to properly diagnose the issue.

Though it is true that for many people who have thyroid conditions, that the right amount of the proper medication will assist in the alleviation of their symptoms, you will have hypothyroidism for the rest of your life if you get it.

To get the best of hypothyroidism it is most commonly treated the best with the use of levothyroxine, also known as Levothroid or Levoxyl, which is T4 put into a synthetic form that is responsible for copying the action the thyroid hormone would regularly take if it were being produced as normal by your body. The idea behind doing this is that the medication will cause a return to the proper levels of the thyroid hormone in your blood. Once a restoration of the thyroid hormone level has occurred, many of the symptoms that come along with having hypothyroidism, will at the very least become much easier to manage, and at best the hypothyroidism symptoms will disappear altogether. It is important to expect it to take several weeks, following treatment, before relief sets in, and you start to feel a return to normalcy. There will also very likely be follow up appointments for testing your blood, which the doctor will recommend in order to keep a solid eye on your progress into recovery. Chances are that you will also receive some medication or other recommended methods to aid you in your recovery, be sure to speak with your doctor about the dosage you should be taking and to come up with a solid plan, that will most benefit you, for recovering in a timely fashion.

It is the case that many people who end up with hypothyroidism medicate for it, for the rest of their lives. Despite this, the dosage you will be taking thru ought that time is likely to go through changes. To better get an idea of how these dosages should be changing over time, it is best to get a check up on your thyroid-stimulation hormone levels every year. In this way, your doctor will be able to more properly adjust the amount you should be taking, or not taking, based on the blood levels indicated by the thyroid-stimulating hormone tests. Only by doing this regularly, will you and your doctor be able to achieve the recovery program that works best for you.

Plans and programs for this achievement may include medications and other hormone supplementation. Once again, synthetic versions of the hormone you need may be used, as they are a widely used and viable practice to aid in the recovery of hypothyroidism. The synthetic version of the hormone T3 is liothyronine, and T4 in its synthetic medication form is called levothyroxine, both of which act as suitable substitutes for their corresponding hormone.

If it was a deficiency in your iodine intake which caused your specific occurrence of hypothyroidism, it is likely that your doctor will recommend a supplementary form of iodine. Keep in mind to ask your doctor, and get the proper testing before taking anything, but selenium and magnesium supplements have been known to aid heavily in the treatment of hypothyroidism.

The golden ticket to any recovery or treatment is usually diet, and in the case of hypothyroidism, there is no exception. Though this is the case, and diet can be incredibly beneficial in your recovery and treatment, do not expect a change in your diet, doctor recommended or otherwise, to replace the need for a prescribed medication. Foods that are rich in selenium or magnesium such as nuts and seeds like the Brazil nut and sunflower seeds have been shown to be very beneficial additions to any diet to aid in the treatment of hypothyroidism.

Balance in your diet will play an especially important role, as the thyroid gland requires particular amounts of iodine in order to properly reach full functionality. There are foods such as whole grains, vegetables, fruits, and lean meats which can handily accomplish this without the need for iodine supplementation.

And of course, diet is only the beginning, exercise as well comes in as an important slice of the treatment and recovery pie. The muscle and joint pain that coincides with hypothyroidism will more often than not leave one to feel extreme fatigue and depression, both of which can be helped by creating and sticking to a regular work out regime. Though no exercise should be discounted, unless specifically told to avoid certain activities by your doctor, there are certain ones which will prove more beneficial than others for treating the symptoms of hypothyroidism. Low impact workouts such as swimming, riding a bike, doing Pilates or yoga, or even a good brisk walk, have been known to be very helpful low impact work outs that are helpful and easy to work in to a daily routine.

The building up of muscle mass by strength training, lifting weights, sit ups, pushups, and pull-ups, help reduce the lethargic feeling of sluggishness that comes along with hypothyroidism. The increase in muscle mass will result in an increase in the rate of your metabolism, which will simultaneously assist in decreasing any weight gain that the hypothyroidism may have caused.

And finally doing training that is primarily cardiovascular. As stated earlier, hypothyroidism is one of the ailments that can correlate with a heightened risk of having a cardiac arrythmia, or irregularity of the heartbeat. By taking steps to be more mindful of your cardiovascular health, exercising on a regular basis or schedule, will help in protecting your heart.

There are also alternative treatments which exist to help in taking care of hypothyroidism, such as animal extracts that contain the thyroid hormone. These extracts are made available from pigs because they contain both the thyroid hormone T4 and thyroid hormone T3. It is uncommon for these to be recommended, however, as they have not shown to be reliable in how to dose, as well as not being more effective than the typically recommended medications. It is also popular to find some glandular extracts in stores that are health food based. The risk that comes along with them is that the U.S. Food and Drug Administration plays no role in the monitoring or the regulation of these extracts. This has historically brought the guarantee of their pureness, legitimacy, and even their potency into question. If you decide to use these products, you do so at your own risk, but still be sure to inform your doctor so that they can adjust accordingly to your treatment.

You can go above and beyond in regards to hypothyroidism treatment, yet still deal with issues or complications that are longer lasting because of this harsh fluctuation to your body. Luckily there have been methods developed and used which will help to lessen the burden of hypothyroidisms effects on your life moving forward.

In the beginning, fatigue can feel like a lot to deal with, especially when associated with depression. These feelings can creep through even if you are taking proper dosages of your medication. It is of utmost importance that you get a good quality sleep every night to ease your treatment and recovery. A good, healthy diet, as well as the relief of stress through activities such as meditation, Pilates, and yoga, are effective strategies when it comes to combating lower energy levels.

It is also vitally important to recognize the difficulty of having a medical condition that is chronic, especially in the case of something like hypothyroidism, which comes along with its own mixed bag of other concerns to your overall health. Being able to talk about, or express, the experience of going through this will help. There are resources out there for support groups of other people who live with the effects of hypothyroidism, you can find a therapist to talk to, perhaps a close friend or loved one. Anyone who will be able to enable you to discuss your experience with openness and with honesty. You may even be able to receive a recommendation for meetings of people with hypothyroidism, from an education office at your local hospital. Connecting and communicating with others who can empathize with what you are going through could end up being an enormous aid in your recovery and life with hypothyroidism.

Important as well is making sure you monitor yourself for other health conditions that could arise. As we went over earlier, the main cause for hypothyroidism is an autoimmune disease. Just as well, links with hypothyroidism have also been found in conditions such as diabetes, having pituitary issues, having your sleep obstructed by sleep apnea, and lupus.

Just as with fatigue, depression is a common symptom and side effect of going through and living with hypothyroidism and should be watched closely. The thyroid glands hormone levels lower, the function of your body begins to slow down, and before you may realize it you are living with a depression that was not there before. It is vital to know what to look out for, and not just what, but also how to look after yourself while dealing with this.

Depression as a symptom can make hypothyroidism difficult to diagnose as there are many who may only experience difficulties or changes in mood as a symptom. It is for this reason, that instead of having a doctor check only your brain when checking for depression, it can also be important to ask them to check for signs of you having an underactive thyroid. Aside from the changes in mood, there are a few other similarities that exist in both having depression as well as hypothyroidism such as, gaining weight, finding it difficult to maintain concentration, feelings of daily fatigue, which coincide with a reduced desire and satisfaction with daily life, and hypothyroidism or depression could both effect your ability to sleep well.

Not all of their symptoms overlap so nicely though, both have their conditions which differentiate one from the other. In the case of hypothyroidism there are, of course, some physical signs such as the dryness of the skin, or the thinning and loss of hair. There is also the tendency to become constipated and the increase in levels of cholesterol. These symptoms would be atypical if depression alone was the issue.

If you have hypothyroidism and it is the cause of your depression, then the correct treatment and care of the hypothyroidism should be just the remedy needed in order to treat your depression as well. If the hypothyroidism passes and depression remains, it may be important to talk to your doctor about receiving further help and a change in medication.

Along with depression being a symptom of hypothyroidism, it has recently been found, through studies, that around 60 percent or so of people who get hypothyroidism tend to also exhibit having anxiety as well. Studies are ongoing and are still growing in scope and size, though it would still be in your best interest to discuss all possibilities and symptoms with your doctor in order to more thoroughly and best tackle the treatment of hypothyroidism.

It cannot be stressed enough, how much of your body is under the affects and influence of your thyroid gland working properly to produce and secrete the correct levels of hormones. For this reason, when a woman gets hypothyroidism and simultaneously desires to get pregnant, she will be faced with her own subset of challenges to come. Have a low thyroid gland function during a pregnancy can cause a number of conflicts including various birth defects, have a still-birth or miscarriage, as well as anemia or a low birth weight. It is not uncommon for a woman with thyroid problems to have a perfectly healthy pregnancy, but to make sure that you reach this outcome it is important to do things such as eating well, keeping yourself informed about current and effective medicines, as well as talking to your doctor about testing.

Though testing may result in changes to your dosage or medication, it is also for this reason that it is important to make sure you are not deviating from the medications provided and the dosage your doctor has recommended.

Considering the thyroid issues adds on even more importance to the need for eating healthy while pregnant. Make sure that you are getting the proper amount of vitamins, minerals, and nutrients and consider taking multivitamins as well to supplement this.

It is not impossible to develop a thyroid issue such as hypothyroidism while pregnant. In fact, for every 1,000 pregnancies, this tends to occur in every 3 out of 5 women. It is important for doctors to routinely check thyroid levels during your pregnancy, as some will do, to make sure your thyroid levels aren't becoming to high or low. If they end up being higher or lower than they ought to be, it is likely that your doctor will recommend you starting treatment. Even some women who have never before had any thyroid issues may develop them once the baby is born, which is known as postpartum thyroiditis, and also tends to resolve itself after a year in around 80 percent of the women it shows up in. It is only the other 20 percent of women who will have this happen and then go on to require the long term treatment.

When hypothyroidism takes place, and the functions of the body slow down, it is quite typical for people to become prone to gaining weight, which is very likely due to what happens to the bodies ability to burn energy, which is that the efficiency to do so slows down as well. This change in the body will typically cause someone who has hypothyroidism to gain anywhere from 5 to 10 pounds in general, making the weight that is gained not entirely drastic, but someone could still find it quite alarming. It is very possible then, that once the hypothyroidism has been treated, that any weight gained will then be easily lost. If this does not occur, a simple change in diet, and adding regular exercise to your routine should aid in handily losing the weight, as your ability to manage weight will go back to normalcy, with the return to proper levels in your thyroid hormones.

Hypothyroidism is a common occurrence; therefore it is also commonly treated without issue. Hypothyroidism has been found to occur in around 4.6 percent of the American population that are 12 and older. Which comes out to about 10 million or so people who go on to live long healthy lives with the condition, and you may never even realize it. It is far more prevalent in people who are over the age of 60, and in women about 1 in 5 of them are likely to experience hypothyroidism by the time they have reached 60 years of age. One of the causes is Hashimoto's disease which happens to appear more in women who have reached middle-age, though it can absolutely show up in children and men. As Hashimoto's disease is hereditary, it is likely that if you get it, you did so from a relative, and have an increased chance then of passing it on down to your children.

It is important to keep an eye on your body, your health, and your thyroid gland as you get older. If, as the years go by, you begin to notice any of the changes gone over in this chapter so far, it is vital that you see a doctor in an attempt to get a proper diagnosis and seek treatment as soon as possible.

Hashimoto's Disease

Hashimoto's disease is an autoimmune disease which can be very destructive to your thyroid gland, and thereby your thyroid glands ability to function properly. Hashimoto's disease is also known as chronic autoimmune lymphocytic thyroiditis and is the most common cause of having an underactive thyroid gland, hypothyroidism, in the United States.

As an autoimmune disorder, Hashimoto's disease is one of many conditions that will be the cause of your body's white blood cells and your body's antibodies becoming confused and starting to attack the cells that make up the thyroid gland. What makes this happen precisely is still somewhat of a mystery to doctors, even still it is believed by some that factors of genetics may be involved.

With the cause of Hashimoto's disease being unknown, it is difficult to precisely put a finger on what puts a person at risk for having or contracting the disease. There are still, however, just a few factors that doctors are aware of which could signify being at risk for the disease. In the case of Hashimoto's disease, in particular, women happen to be seven times more likely to contract than men, and especially for women who have been pregnant before. Having a history of autoimmune diseases in the family is another factor that could mean you are at higher risk of having Hashimoto's at some point in your life, especially if the autoimmune diseases include Graves' disease, lupus, rheumatoid arthritis, if there is a history of Sjogren's syndrome in your family, or a history of type 1 diabetes, Addison's disease, and vitiligo. If it is the case that these autoimmune diseases are present in your family line or may have been based on symptoms of Hashimoto's disease, get together and discuss the possibility with your doctor, then make sure to get tested for the disease.

Hashimoto's disease is interesting in that the symptoms of it, are not symptomatic of Hashimoto's disease alone, in fact, they are similar to having the symptoms of an underactive thyroid gland, or hypothyroidism. Some signs to watch out for that your thyroid gland is not working properly to produce proper thyroid hormones, and that you may have Hashimoto's disease are your skin becoming dry and pale, constipation, if your voice becomes hoarse, you become depressed and start to feel sluggish or fatigued. High levels of cholesterol, a thinning of the hair, muscle weakness in the lower body, and intolerance to the cold may also be signs of hypothyroidism as a result of Hashimoto's disease. In women, it can also cause issues with fertility. Hashimoto's can exist inside of your body for many years before you begin to show any signs or symptoms, and during that time, it may progress while showing no signs of damage to the thyroid gland. Some with Hashimoto's disease end up with a goiter, an enlarging of the thyroid gland which causes the front of the neck to swell. Though generally painless, it is common for a goiter to make the act of swallowing difficult and for it to simulate a feeling of fullness in the throat.

Owing to it's difficulty to diagnose, your doctor may not suspect Hashimoto's of being prevalent until observing symptoms having hypothyroidism. In which case they will need to conduct a blood test designed to check the thyroid-stimulating hormone, or TSH, levels in your body. It is a relatively common and safe test, which is also an accurate way to check to see if you have Hashimoto's disease. Levels of thyroid-stimulating hormone are higher when the activity of the thyroid glad is lower because your body starts working harder to stimulate the production of more thyroid hormones to secrete from the thyroid gland. There are also blood tests that your doctor may conduct if they feel the need to check further for the levels of antibodies, cholesterol, and other thyroid hormones, T3 and T4, in your blood. Testing for all of these can help immensely in pinning down a diagnosis of Hashimoto's disease.

Unless your thyroid gland is functioning normally, in which case your doctor may still recommend regular checkups to monitor you for any changes, it is very likely that the need for treatment of Hashimoto's disease will be required.

The improper production of enough hormones in your body by your thyroid gland will likely result in the need to take medication. In the case of having to take this medication, it is also likely that you will be prescribed on it, though dose will vary, for the rest of your life. The effective drug most commonly prescribed is levothyroxine which is the hormone thyroxine, or T4, made synthetically, and which will successfully replace the missing hormone in your blood. The synthetic hormone drug levothyroxine tends not to have any noticeable side effects, and regular use has been known to frequently return the hormone levels of the body back to normal, restoring proper function of the thyroid gland. When this happens, all other symptoms of Hashimoto's disease and hypothyroidism generally tend to disappear altogether, though it is likely that your doctor will still recommend that you still get regular testing done so that your hormone levels can be consistently monitored to prevent something like hypothyroidism from becoming a problem again moving forward. Getting the regular testing allows the doctor to adjust the dosage of your medication as necessary if at all necessary.

It is important to consider before going on levothyroxine, that there are supplements and medications which will have an effect on your body's ability to absorb the drug. As such, make sure you have a discussion about this with your doctor if you are taking any other medications, especially if they include iron or calcium supplements, or estrogen. Some medications for cholesterol have been known to cause an issue, as well as proton pump inhibitors which are used as a treatment for acid reflux.

Though these have been known to cause an issue, there is what could be an easy work around of simply changing what time of the day you take your other medicines in conjunction with the doctor recommended thyroid medicine. It is also possible that certain foods could end up being involved in the efficacy of your thyroid medicine. It is best to discuss all of this with your doctor to come up with an efficient way for you to take your thyroid medicine, based on your dietary needs.

The severity of complications due to leaving Hashimoto's untreated varies and are not worth the risk if you ever contract, or if you have it. They go far beyond just hypothyroidism and include heart problems that an include total failure of the heart. It is not unusual for anemia to be a result of leaving Hashimoto's disease unattended. Depression and a decrease in libido are common, as well as higher levels of cholesterol in the blood and experiencing a sense of confusion or loss of consciousness.

Hashimoto's disease has also been the culprit responsible for complications during a woman's pregnancy cycle. It is far more likely, that if you carry out a pregnancy while having untreated Hashimoto's disease, that you may be putting your child at higher risk of being born with defects of their kidneys, their heart, and even their brains.

These complications can be limited by talking to your doctor during the pregnancy and keeping on top of monitoring your thyroid glands hormone levels with the proper blood testing. If you are a pregnant woman and have thyroid issues, such preventative measures could mean a severe change in the life and health of your child. However, if you have not had any known disorders with your thyroid or hormone levels, it is not recommended that you get regular or constant screening done during the pregnancy.

Graves' Disease

Another autoimmune disorder, Graves' disease is responsible for causing your thyroid gland too create too much of the thyroid hormones in your body. When this happens it is a condition referred to commonly as hyperthyroidism. Graves' disease, is named such for the man who discovered it, an Irish physician named Robert J. Graves, and is regarded as one of the most common forms hyperthyroidism takes, having an effect on around 1 out of every 200 people.

When Graves' disease occurs in the body, it will cause your immune system to begin creating antibodies that are known as thyroid-stimulating immunoglobulins, that attach themselves to the body's usually healthy cells of the thyroid gland. By doing this they end up causing the thyroid gland to produce and secrete more of the thyroid hormones than it is meant to for your body. The hormones that are produced by the thyroid gland go on to affect a great number of your body's functions including its temperature, the function of the nervous system, the development of the brain, and the list goes on. For this reason, hyperthyroidism can end up having a negatively driven affect on not just all of those functions, but when left untreated can also cause the loss of weight and mental and physical fatigue. Hyperthyroidism has also been found to be responsible for such things as depression and emotional liability where the individual will uncontrollably cry or laugh or put on other manic emotional displays.

Due to the role that Graves' disease can invariably play on the appearance of hyperthyroidism in the body, it is no surprise that the two would contain a sharing of many of the same symptoms. These symptoms include tremors especially of the hands, a loss of weight, tachycardia, which is the rapidity in the rate of the heart, becoming intolerant to heat or warmth, fatigue, nervousness and irritability, the swelling of the front of the neck, due to the enlargement of the thyroid gland, known as a goiter, an increase in the frequency of having bowel movements, as well as diarrhea, weakness of the muscles, and having it become difficult to get a good full night's worth of sleep. Among the people who experience having Graves' disease, it is only a small percentage who will experience the skin thickening around their shin area and become reddened, an affliction which is known as Graves' dermopathy.

Another common symptom of Graves' disease which one may go through while experiencing the condition, is what is called Graves' ophthalmopathy. Graves' ophthalmopathy is what occurs when the eyes of the afflicted individual appear to be enlarged, which is a result of the eyelids retracting. When Graves' ophthalmopathy happens, it is entirely possible that your eyes may begin to bulge outwards from your eye sockets. Estimates say that as much as 30 percent of the people who end up developing Graves' disease will observe at least a mild case of what is known as Graves' ophthalmopathy and that for up to 5 percent of the people will instead experience an extreme case of the eye bulging.

Because of autoimmune diseases such as Graves' disease, the immune system will begin to fight against what are the healthy cells and healthy tissues of the body. Normally, your immune system is producing proteins which are known as antibodies, which are responsible for fighting against foreign invaders to your body, the likes of harmful viruses and bacteria. The antibodies produced this way are formed especially with the duty of targeting a specific invader to the host. When it comes to the effect of Graves' disease on the body, your immune system begins to mistake healthy thyroid cells as these foreign harmful cells and produces the thyroid-stimulating immunoglobulins which then mistakenly go off to attack what are your healthy thyroid cells.

Scientists and doctors alike, are aware that it is indeed possible for a person to have inherited the ability for their body to make antibodies which then go against their own healthy cells, yet they have made no determination that such an occurrence is what is the cause for Graves' disease, or who will end up developing Graves' disease.

Despite that though, there are experts who believe that they have been able to button down on some factors which may increase ones risk for the development of graves disease which includes its tendency to be hereditary. So be sure to discuss family medical history with your doctor and talk about whether or not there are family members who have, or who ay have had Graves' disease. It is also believed by these experts that stress, gender, and someone's age may be some of the facets that end up putting someone at higher risk of getting Graves' disease. It is typical for the disease to be found in people who are younger than the age of 40, and it has been more prevalent, about seven to eight times so, in women rather than men.

Having had, or having still, another autoimmune disease is yet another factor that will increase your risk of ever getting Graves' disease. Examples of such autoimmune diseases are having Crohn's disease, rheumatoid arthritis, and diabetes mellitus, among others.

For the diagnosing of Graves' disease, when it is suspected, it is not unheard of for your doctor to request lab tests. The use of your families medical history as well, especially if there is a case of someone in your family having had Graves' disease, will be able to help act as a basis for your doctor to zero in on diagnosing whether you have Graves' disease as well or not. This is something that thyroid gland blood tests will be needed for in order to confirm. Your doctor may request that these tests and others may be handled by a specialist expert in diseases which are related to the body's hormones, known as an endocrinologist, in order to help get the diagnosis of Graves' disease. Other tests which your doctor may request are full bloodwork tests, a thyroid gland scan, an uptake test utilizing radioactive iodine, a test for levels of TSH, or thyroid stimulating hormone, and a TSI test, which is the thyroid-stimulating immunoglobulins.

By combining the efforts of the endocrinologist, as well as the array of tests, it is more possible for your doctor to determine if you do indeed have and need treatment for Graves' disease specifically, or if another thyroid disorder is what is at work, and thus requires its own specific form of treatment.

There are a number of options available for treatment when someone is diagnosed as having Graves' disease. These are generally the taking of anti-thyroid drugs, therapy in the form of RAI, or radioactive iodine, and getting thyroid gland surgery. It is not abnormal for a doctor, in the case of Graves' disease, to recommend, all, two, or just one of the treatments for the afflicted.

When it comes to treatment via anti-thyroid drugs, you will typically be taking medications such as methimazole, which is taken orally as a tablet and works by putting a stop to the thyroid gland producing and secreting too much thyroid hormone, and propylthiouracil, which is also taken orally and generally used as a back up if a drug like methimazole did not end up working well enough. The use of beta-blockers is also recommended on occasion as they are used in assistance of reducing the effects of symptoms until another treatment method can start working.

It is radioactive iodine treatment, or RAI, which is among the most common treatments suggested to those suffering of Graves' disease. It is required, during this treatment, that the individual seeking treatment take specified doses of radioactive iodine-131, the purpose of which is to destroy thyroid cells. The radioactive iodine-131 will be ingested orally, in small amounts, via pill. Be sure to discuss with your doctor and risks or precautions that come with this treatment.

The less frequent option for treatment is the thyroid surgery. This treatment will tend to be a last resort if the other options have not worked to full capacity, if there is a reason to be suspect of thyroid cancer being present, or if the patient is a pregnant woman who is unable to take any of the regularly prescribed anti-thyroid drugs.

In the case of surgery being necessary, it is not uncommon the doctor to issue the removal of your thyroid gland completely, in the interest of preventing the return of the hyperthyroidism. In which case, thyroid hormone replacement surgery will be necessary on a regular basis. Talk to your doctor about the possible side effects of choosing to go through with surgery, as well as generally what to expect moving forward.

Goiter

A goiter, goitre, thyroid cyst, or Plummer's disease, is a general term used for when there is an observable enlargement of the thyroid gland, usually resulting in a noticeable swelling of the front of the neck. Treatment for a goiter can be handled in a variety of ways, and the treatment method is dependent on the goiters location, the length of its presence, and how exactly it is affecting the thyroid glands performance.

Though usually unable to be seen or even felt, the thyroid gland generally tends to become detectable by touch and even perceptible to the eye when there is a goiter present. An expanse of the thyroid gland, or goiter, can be the cause of the whole thyroid gland expanding, which is known as a "smooth goiter", or just a part of the thyroid gland expanding, which is also called a "cystic" or "nodular" goiter. A goiter is not a sure symptom of having an active thyroid, known as hyperthyroidism, or underactive thyroid, known as hypothyroidism, and, in fact, the majority of people who have a goiter, retain a perfectly normal use of their thyroid gland.

A number of reasons exist for the existence of a goiter. Among these are included a deficiency in your levels of iodine. Iodine may be a trace element, but it is far from trivial. It assists in helping the thyroid gland in maintaining proper functionality and making the thyroid glands hormones. There are two primary hormones which are produced and secreted by the thyroid gland, these are T4 or thyroxine, and T3, also known as triiodothyronine. The approximate number of people who have iodine deficiency comes out to about 2.2 billion and it is estimated that around 29 percent of the worlds total population live in an area that is considered to be deficient in iodine. It is reported that people in the U.K. have proper levels of iodine as a part of their regular diet. If you are keeping your eye out for food sources that are a good source of iodine, there are salts that have iodine supplements, as well, non-organic milk is plentiful with iodine.

Thyroiditis is anther well known cause of goiter. Thyroiditis is more commonly referred to as when the thyroid gland has become inflamed. Around the world, the most common reason for thyroiditis occurring is Hashimoto's disease, or Hashimoto's thyroiditis, which is an autoimmune disease that causes the bodies antibodies to start to become confused and begin attacking healthy cells of the thyroid gland. Hashimoto's disease is not the only cause of the thyroiditis condition though, it could also stem from viral infection, and has been known to occur just after or during pregnancy.

A goiter has also been known to occur due to Graves' disease, another autoimmune disease, this one causing the immune systems antibodies attacks on thyroid cells to make the thyroid gland overactive, resulting in hyperthyroidism. It is this hyperthyroidism, or over activity of the thyroid glands capacity for producing and secreting hormones, which is the cause of the swelling of the thyroid gland.

If there are benign growths on the thyroid gland, they have been known to cause a goiter, most commonly known for doing this is a follicular adenoma, which can be a firm or rubbery tumor surrounded by a fibrous capsule.

External factors that may be the cause of goiter are known as goitrogens. Included among what would be considered a goitrogen are medicines such as the mental health drug lithium, and cabbage type vegetables. Ingestion in the excess of these vegetables, which include cassava or kelp, will likely result in the growth formation of a goiter.

There are physiological demands put on the body during pregnancy and during puberty which have been known to be at the root of a goiter. And as with other causes like Graves' disease and Hashimoto's disease, there is a strong likelihood of inherited genetic reasons that one may at some point experience goiter.

Due to the varying reasons for the existence of goiter, there are also a multiplicity of types of goiter. The first of these types is known as colloid goiter, or endemic goiter, which is a development due directly to a lack of sufficient iodine levels. As a result, the people who tend to end up with a colloid goiter are those we mentioned, who live somewhere with a less dense supply of iodine.

The next type of goiter is the nontoxic goiter, or sporadic goiter, as it is also well known. Though the definite cause of a goiter of this type is regarded as generally unknown, it is surmised that a sporadic goiter is a result of taking medications, such as lithium, for example, or so it is believed. Among the may uses for lithium, it is perhaps most commonly recognized as the drug used for aiding in the treatment of mood based disorders, the likes of bipolar or depression. The nontoxic name is apt in regard to this form of goiter, as they are benign, and have no discernable effect on the production or secretion function of the thyroid gland, leaving the thyroid to function at a healthy and normal capacity.

The final type of commonly recognized goiter is known as the toxic nodular or multinodular goiter. Generally originating and taking form from as merely an extension from what was a simple goiter prior, the toxic nodular goiter will take the form of at least one, but often more, small nodules on the expanding thyroid gland. This toxic nodular goiter, having taken a sort of root on the thyroid gland, then begins to produce its own thyroid hormone, which plays a big part in the causation of hyperthyroidism.

As mentioned above, it can be difficult to detect goiter before it has really taken effect to the thyroid gland, but after it has begun doing it's work it is most common for it to cause a swelling of the front of the neck, making it clearly visible as well as felt. Before the expanding has commenced, it is common to have had nodules existing in your thyroid gland, these small nodules cannot be felt, and may have even been only a chance occurrence due to examinations, and of scans, that were applied for other reasons. Cases such as these are rather common, and when they occur, there has been a tendency to notice no sign of a goiter up to that point. As nodules appear on the thyroid, ranging from smaller nodules to much larger nodules, it is the presence of these nodules which is what is the cause of noticeable swelling of the neck.

This swelling and the nodules which are collecting on the thyroid gland cause other symptoms to occur, like having a difficult time of swallowing or of trying to breathe, it is not uncommon for coughing to be a symptom, your voice may start to become hoarse, and there may be a dizzy sensation that is noticeable when you raise an arm above your head.

Goiter is a rather common occurrence. It is calculated by the World Health Organization, that around the world, goiter affects nearly 12 percent of the global population. However, it has also been recorded that in Europe, the rate of goiter is lower by a slight amount. Goiter being considered endemic, or noticeably affecting a certain area is a common occurrence wherever iodine is scarce, and the endemic definitions are only applied when goiter is recognized on 1 out of 10 people within a certain population.

It is usual for goiter to be the diagnosis when there is noticeable swelling on the neck that can be seen without the need of a scan, also making it detectable with the touch of the hand, due to the enlarged thyroid gland in your neck, something a doctor will be quick to check for, likely before anything else.

There are also a number tests a general practitioner may order in order to examine the levels in your blood of thyroid hormones coming from the thyroid gland, as well as wanting to make sure of the levels of antibodies that are prevalent in the bloodstream. This examination will often take the form of blood tests, that are used to detect the changes in levels of the hormones as well as whether or not the level of production of the antibodies has increased, which tends to happen in response to the body experiencing an injury or infection in the blood.

A thyroid scan, or thyroid uptake scan, will show the size of the goiter itself, as well as what condition the goiter is in. It will also aid in identifying any differences in activity, in various places on the thyroid gland.

A biopsy may be recommended, the procedure of which involves removing samples of your thyroid gland, and then sending the samples of your thyroid gland's tissue to an outside laboratory or endocrinologist for examination.

It is also possible that an ultrasound scan may be used which will help for a doctor to see images of the inside of your neck, getting a much closer look at the size of the invasive goiter, allowing for the observation of nodules. As more ultrasounds are done, it is even then possible to track the changes in size or shape of the nodules, and the size of the goiter.

You may, at some point, be referred to an endocrinologist in order to get an outpatient assessment, giving you and the doctor more information from the examination by an expert. During their examination you may have to undergo a test known as a fine needle aspiration, which is done on the thyroid gland. For the procedure to take place, the endocrinologist will make use of a fine needle which, utilizing the guiding sight of an ultrasound, will be used to remove tissue from your thyroid gland, only a small amount will be needed. The tissue removed from your thyroid gland is then studied under the lens of a microscope, which will assist the endocrinologist in assessing exactly the types of cells which are currently present in your thyroid gland. It is not at all uncommon for a procedure like this to need to be repeated one or more times, for the sake of reaching an accurate result and helping you on your way to treatment and recovery.

There is no one, cut and dry, blanket method for treating a goiter, as the treatment will depend entirely on precisely what is the cause that is underlying the goiter. As well, a particular course of action will be decided by your doctor on the basis of the size of the goiter, and the condition that the goiter is in, as well as the symptoms you have that are associated with the goiter. It will also be important to not overlook any factors to your health that may have been responsible for the goiters formation when looking into treatment options.

A goiter which can be regarded as simple, having a prevalence of causing no imbalances in the thyroid gland, as well as no seeming problems as a result of the thyroid gland, will be less likely to cause further obstructions or overall issues.

In order to shrink a goiter, in the case of hypo or hyperthyroidism, it may be enough to just take prescribed medicines as a treatment for the symptoms and for the swelling of the thyroid gland. Medications which are known as corticosteroids often see use in the task of reducing any inflammation, or when there is a prevalence of thyroiditis.

Medicinal treatments for a goiter are not always the most effective response, however. It is not at all uncommon for a goiter to have grown too large to be able to respond properly to medicinal therapy and begin to shrink. In such a case there are surgeries which are available, known as a thyroidectomy. Undergoing a thyroidectomy will mean removing your thyroid gland completely and is a common option for when the thyroid gland grows too large and further obstructs what would otherwise be simple actions, such as swallowing or breathing.

When you are going through the experience of trying to treat what is the most harmful of the goiter family, the toxic nodular or multinodular goiter, RAI, or radioactive iodine treatment is typically the necessary response. You will be given a tablet, the RAI, which is a small amount of the radioactive iodine, which gets ingested orally and begins the process of destroying thyroid gland tissue.

When it comes to the treatment of a goiter, there are options for home care which can be very helpful and ought not to be overlooked as such. When you have finished up with all the treatment that can be offered at the hospital, or by a referred endocrinologist, it is an entirely common possibility that a discussion with your general practitioner will end in him or her suggesting you continue care of yourself in the home, with a prescription of some form of medication, which may end up being a decrease or increase in the amounts of iodine that you are ingesting regularly. This will, of course, be determined by the type of goiter that was ailing you, as well as requiring regular testing to keep an eye on your iodine levels, and the efficiency of your thyroid glands production and secretion of hormones. If it all ends up that a goiter is non-problematic, being too small to count as an issue or cause an imbalance, you may require no treatment or care at home at all.

PART 2

Chapter 1: What is the Alkaline Diet

We eat the foods that we eat for all kinds of different reasons. Sure, from an evolutionary standpoint, we eat food so that we can take in calories and convert them into energy in order to fuel our bodies and keep us going throughout the entire day. The food we eat also provides us with the essential nutrients that our bodies need in order to keep them running in an optimal manner.

But we also eat food for pleasure, the sheer joy of tasting something amazing that we truly love. We eat socially. Food has been a way of bringing people together since the very dawn of civilization. Sometimes we use food for comfort and sometimes we use it to mark formal and important occasions. We use food as a proving ground over which to test out new prospective romantic partners.

And yet, for all that food can do for us, so many of us take it for granted and don't seek out ways to make our food work for us. Used correctly, food and nutrition are tools that can turn our bodies into the healthiest and efficient powerhouse that nature intended them to be.

With so many different diets and nutrition plans out there, it can be hard to know which one is right for you. Well, you're reading this book so you already know that you're on the right track!

Indeed, the alkaline diet is a tried and tested way to get the most out of your body. But how does it work? Why does it work? How can eating an alkaline diet optimize your body and health?

The key to understanding the science and chemistry behind how the foods we eat affect us is to understand that just like the fundamental laws of physics, every action has an equal and opposite reaction. Or in other words, everything that we put into our bodies will affect us based on the characteristics of that particular food item. So if we eat a lot of things that cause the same or similar effects on our bodies, we can influence and even control the effects and changes that our body takes by carefully selecting the foods that we eat and what effect they have on our bodies. As the popular saying goes — you are what you eat.

To illustrate, imagine you are walking through the woods and you accidentally brush up against a poison ivy leaf. Well, sorry to say it, but there is a very good chance that you are going to develop an itchy poison ivy rash. If however, you get completely naked and roll around in an entire patch of poison ivy, you are pretty much guaranteed to get poison ivy and a whole lot of it!

Humorous examples aside, it stands to reason that if we know that a particular food or food group has a particular effect on our body, we can effectively control any number of internal body systems by carefully planning and selecting the foods we eat.

So how does the alkaline diet promote health? Well, the alkaline diet is all about balance. So many of the negative health issues in our lives are the result of an imbalance in our bodies. So much of the history of medicine revolves around finding the ideal balances for the human body.

For many, many years, doctors around the world attributed all of our health conditions, whether good or ill, to a balance or imbalance in what they referred to as the "humors". As far back as Ancient Greece and Ancient Rome, there was a near-universal belief that four humors or bodily fluids influenced every aspect of health and temperament, and ill health or ill temperament was the result of deficiencies or excesses on one or more of these four humors. These four humors were black bile, yellow bile, phlegm, and blood. Each of these four humors was associated with a particular personality type and other such characteristics.

When a person came to an ancient doctor with an ailment, the ancient doctor would examine their patient to determine their temperament and along with other factors would determine where their imbalance in humors was, and then they would come up with a treatment plan with the intention of balancing the patient's humors. So in other words, for millennia, the goal of medicine has been to achieve balance in the human body.

And while many of the theories and practices of ancient physicians have long ago fallen out of use in favor of new techniques and schools of thought, modern science has nevertheless confirmed at least some aspects of ancient medicine, namely, the concept of balance itself.

While we don't hear much about black bile, yellow bile, or phlegm anymore in modern medicine, the fourth humor that ancient doctors treated is certainly still extremely prominent in modern medicine — blood.

Blood is still very much our life force just as it was believed by ancient doctors. Blood is the fluid that keeps us living and breathing and a proper medical understanding is absolutely integral to maintain overall good health.

So how can we maintain a good balance in our blood? What aspect of our blood do we even need to balance? What negative effects can we avoid by maintaining balanced blood and what positive ones can we promote?

While those ancient doctors were certainly on the right track, they had a few key factors wrong so, in order to move forward, we are going to need a firmer and more modern grasp of the science behind our health and nutrition.

To understand this concept a little bit better, we need to understand one of the most fundamental aspects of chemistry. This integral part of chemistry and science as a whole is known as the pH balance or the pH scale. We are going to learn all about the pH balance or the pH scale and how it can affect our bodies in a positive way in the following chapters. First, we will learn what a pH balance is.

Chapter 2: What is a pH Balance?

The first thing we need to understand on our journey to the perfect internal balance via the alkaline diet is exactly just what the pH balance is. Furthermore, we need to understand how the chemical characteristics of a substance or fluid play a role in determining where it falls on the pH scale.

What exactly does the pH scale measure? In short, the pH scale is a measure of the acidity or basicity of solution in which the solvent is water. Such a solution is known as an aqueous solution. In other words, when a substance is dissolved in or is otherwise mixed with water, it can then be tested and measured on the pH scale.

An aqueous solution can be defined as either an acid or a base, as this is precisely what the pH scale is meant to determine. An aqueous solution that is basic is referred to as being alkaline. This gives us a pretty good indication of what the alkaline diet is all about. The pH scale itself is a type of scale known as a logarithmic scale. This means that each equidistant quantified measure is an order of magnitude greater than the previous measurement on the scale. The scale ranges from zero to fourteen, with a neutral pH value being in the middle at seven.

Solutions that have a pH value of less the median value of seven are defined as being acidic, while the opposite scenario, in which a solution is measured to have a pH value of higher than seven — that solution is called basic. Water that is pure and unadulterated is pH neutral which is to say that it should prove to have a pH value of seven when tested, as natural dihydrogen oxide, the chemical name for water is neither a base nor an acid. If that is not the case, then the water should be tested for impurities.

While it is possible for an aqueous solution to have a pH value greater than fourteen or less than zero, these would have to be extremely acidic or extremely basic solutions and would not only be decisively deadly to ingest and even extremely dangerous just to touch. Therefore, for practical purposes, official pH values are nearly always represented on a scale between zero and fourteen.

The pH scale is defined by a set of international standards that are determined and agreed upon by an international scientific body. There are several ways to test the pH level of an aqueous solution, with one of the most notable ones being the use of a glass electrode combined with a pH meter. This scientific instrument determines the difference between a pH electrode and a control electrode in terms of their respective electrical potential. This difference in the electrical potential of a solution relates directly to the acidity of the solution and can therefore be used to give it a standard value.

Another very popular and frequently used means by which to test the pH value of an aqueous solution is by using one of the various compounds known as pH indicators.

A pH indicator is generally some kind of substance that when mixed with an aqueous solution results in a chemical reaction that will literally change the color of the solution, and by examining and comparing the color of the resulting solution, the pH value of the solution can be determined. There are other pH indicators that indicate the pH level of a solution by chemical reactions that result in other physical indicators such as odor for example. However, by far the most common variety of pH indicators are visual in nature, generally based around color.

One of the most common types of pH indicators is the naturally occurring family of chemical compounds called anthocyanin. These compounds naturally change color reflects the pH balance of whatever item the compound is found within. Generally, these compounds are found in colored plant leaves or other plant parts. One of the most common sources of these pH indicating compounds is from the leaves of a red cabbage. The reason for this is because it is quite easy to extract anthocyanin from a red cabbage making it the perfect resource for a homemade pH indicator test for either health or educational purposes.

Anthocyanin can be found in many different plants though, such as the leaves of the aforementioned red cabbage, but also in certain flowers such as the geranium, the poppy, and also rose petals. Berries and stems can also house anthocyanin compounds such as blueberries and blackcurrants as well as rhubarb. In short, most plants or vegetables that have reddish, purplish, or bluish color in all likelihood contain at least a small amount of anthocyanin compound. When used as a pH indicator by mixing it with an aqueous solution, an anthocyanin compound will become redder the more acidic the solution is and will turn from red to purple to blue the more alkaline the solution is.

Another very commonly used pH indicator since medieval times is the substance called litmus which is derived from various species of lichen. In fact, the word litmus itself means colored moss in its original language, Old

Norse. Just like anthocyanin compounds, litmus will turn red when exposed to acidic solutions and blue when exposed to basic solutions. You may even be familiar with the term 'litmus test'. It has come to be used very commonly and very broadly as a metaphor for anything that could be used to soundly distinguish between multiple options.

So with pH balance being fundamental to the chemical nature of all kinds of biological material including the foods we eat, how do we know if and how such foods are affecting our health? We will continue learning about pH imbalance in our bodies to find out. The next chapter will go into the science of how pH balance or more specifically imbalance can affect our bodies and our health.

Chapter 3: The Science Behind pH Imbalance

Every single substance in the world has a pH balance and that includes all of us. Sure, we don't make cabbages change color when we pick them up, but our bodies must maintain a certain pH level in order to live and function properly. This pH balance that is naturally maintained in our bodies is called the acid-based balance and it is quite literally exactly what it sounds like — the balance of acidic and basic substances in your body. More specifically though, when we are referring to the acid-base balance of our bodies, we are most often referring to the pH balance of our blood.

The human body is designed with a few systems in place intended to keep the natural pH levels regulated at an appropriate balance between acidity and alkalinity. Both the kidneys as well as the lungs have a very important role to play in this process. As we previously laid out, the pH balance is generally expressed as a value between zero and fourteen, with seven being the neutral value. And remember that pure and unadulterated water should have a pH value of exactly seven. Knowing then that water is neutral seven on the pH scale, and knowing also that our bodies are designed to maintain an even pH balance, it would stand to reason that our blood should have a neutral pH value of seven as well, right?

Well, not quite. And this is a major key to understand the alkaline diet. The ideal blood pH level is not actually a neutral seven but instead generally should be about a 7.40 on the pH scale. This value can vary slightly from person to person, but that is the standard average. And yes, that's right— the human body should have a blood pH level that is a little bit on the alkaline side.

Generally speaking, it is the kidneys and lungs that regulate this pH level, so if they are not functioning normally, the blood pH level can become imbalanced. This kind of pH imbalance can lead to serious medical conditions which are called acidosis or alkalosis depending on which direction the imbalance goes in. It is important to note that these serious medical conditions must be treated by a medical professional and diet alone cannot entirely reverse these conditions.

Now, what we're talking about in this book is the small, minor imbalances that a general practitioner wouldn't be concerned about because they aren't severe enough to have a serious debilitating effect, but that certainly do have your body operating in sub-optimal conditions, and more importantly, the alkaline diet that can have it function far better than you ever imagined possible.

So in order to better understand how the alkaline diet will allow us to correct these small but important pH imbalances, we'll need to have a complete understanding of what could throw our pH out of balance and why it might happen.

As we have established a moment ago, the primary regulators of the body's pH level are the kidneys and the lungs. There are a large number of small systems in our bodies that have their own pH level and regulate them in their own ways, but the two main, body-wide regulators are the lungs and kidneys.

As you are likely already aware, we take in oxygen with our lungs when we inhale and expel carbon dioxide when we exhale. The oxygen that we take in is absorbed inside our lungs and used as fuel by our cells. The waste product that our cells produce by using the oxygen is carbon dioxide. Which is all very simple and pretty straightforward and familiar to all of us but here's the important part — carbon dioxide is slightly acidic. So by making slight adjustments to how much carbon dioxide is released or retained, our lungs are able to make adjustments to the overall acid-base level of our blood.

Similarly, the kidneys being the filtration system for the vascular system have the ability to excrete small amounts of acidic or basic compounds into the blood in order to make slight alterations to our blood chemistry. This is a slow process as compared to the more immediate effect of the lungs' pH regulatory system. So the lungs and the kidneys could be thought of as the short-term and long-term blood pH level regulators of our body.

If the blood pH level is out of balance, then it can lead to one of these two conditions — alkalosis and acidosis. With the standard balanced blood pH level being 7.40, anything below 7.35 is considered acidosis and anything above 7.45 is called alkalosis. Again, it is important to note that these are serious medical conditions and must be treated by a medical professional. It is always best to consult your doctor if you are suffering from these conditions. What we can do, however, is assist our body's natural pH regulation system by maintaining a blood pH level that is within the tolerable limits.

A low blood pH level or in other words, slightly acidic blood is far more common than the inverse and so that it is what we are primarily focusing on — an alkaline diet that will help us maintain a healthy blood pH level.

While any level measured at 7.35 and under is acidosis and needs professional medical treatment, it is far too common for our blood pH level to fall into that 'safe' range of 7.36-7.39 without being at that ideal sweet spot of 7.40. If you want to get the most out of your body, if you want your body to be operating at peak performance, and if you want to live your absolute healthiest life, then the 'safe' level of 7.36 is not tolerable for your body.

If you are truly serious about your health and your wellbeing, then the 'safe' blood pH level of 7.39 isn't even good enough for you. You need to have the absolute optimal blood pH level and you will settle for nothing but a perfect 7.40. Continue on reading in the next chapters and we are going to show you how.

Chapter 4: Why Alkaline is Best

If our body's pH level is all about balance, then why would maintaining an alkaline diet be superior to an acidic one? Shouldn't we be consuming a perfect balance of alkaline and acidic foods and nutrition? If those are among the questions you are now asking yourself, then you are on the right track. Those are great questions to ask.

There are several reasons why an alkaline diet is a crucial component in maintaining a healthy body and blood pH level. Remember that magic number? The ideal pH level for our blood that will allow our body to operate optimally? That is right — it was 7.40. And do you remember what the pH value for perfectly pure, unadulterated water is? That is right — it was a perfect seven. So what that means, of course, is that the ideal blood pH balance is in fact slightly alkaline at 0.4 units more basic than water.

So we can see already that in order to maintain our ideal pH balance, we will need to intake more alkaline foods than acidic foods. Of course, that is not to say that you can never consume anything acidic. In fact, it is important to have acids as well in order to maintain balance. We just need to be perfectly aware that our body does in fact require a slight alkaline balance and so we should be mindful of this when we plan our meals and overall diets.

This balance may also be reflected in the foods we choose to eat. They don't necessarily need to be extremely alkaline in order to transfer to us the health benefits we are looking for. They may only need to have a slight pull on the alkaline side of the scale. It all depends on our individual bodies and what they are in need of. And of course, everything scales. So a lot of a slightly alkaline substance may have the same value as a little of something with a higher alkaline value. Remember as well that the pH scale is logarithmic which is to say that each unit is exponential to the value of the previous unit. That means that consuming something with an alkaline value of nine would be ten times more alkaline than something with the alkaline value of eight. This is why we need to be careful when consuming anything that is alkaline or acidic. Things can become unhealthy or even dangerous in a real hurry. So, remember to plan ahead and do everything in moderation.

Another equally surface-level reason why it is important to consume a healthy amount of alkaline rich foods is because whether we are aware of it or not, many if not most of the foods we eat on a regular basis are either slightly or moderately acidic. Some very common foods and beverages even go as far as being highly acidic.

Now, again, it bears repeating that this does not mean that you cannot or should not consume these types of acidic foods and beverages at all. In fact, some of these acidic foods and beverages are very healthy and high in essential nutrients. The important thing, however, is to be aware of how much acidic substances we are consuming and how acidic those substances are.

Do you like fruit juices? How about coffee? Those are two great examples of highly acidic beverages that many of us consume on a regular basis. That is not necessarily a bad thing but just think about this — are you taking in the necessary amount of alkaline foods or liquids in order to maintain a healthy and optimal balance?

And what's more, it can often be a good deal more complicated than whether the particular food item that we are consuming is acidic or alkaline on a surface level. What makes the important difference is how the item we consume affects our blood pH level after it has been metabolized. And that could, in fact, be a good deal different than what it might seem to be based on the original acidity or alkalinity of the food item in question.

Another very important reason to remember to include alkaline foods in our diet in order to maintain a good acid-base blood balance is that an acid rich environment is considered by medical professionals to be a hotbed of disease and illness. And remember, it doesn't take much to become imbalanced in one's blood levels, so even a minor imbalance could quickly become a breeding ground for all manner of illness and health problems that you will absolutely want to avoid.

Just by remembering to consume a healthy and appropriate amount of alkaline foods and drinks, we can be safeguarding ourselves from any number of serious health concerns that could be lurking in our very blood. If you want to kill all of those potential illnesses dead before they become a real concern, you will need to act now and ensure that you are consuming an appropriate amount of alkaline foods.

This is the very topic that we will be going into next. We now know how important it is to maintain a good acid-base blood balance. We now know what that optimal blood pH balance is. And most importantly, we now know the dangers associated with having blood that is too acidic, and why it is so common for us to have a blood pH level that skews a little bit too acidic but not enough to go into full acidosis.

Equipped with this crucial information, we can now move on to learning about how to apply these factors to our everyday lives. Now, we are going to learn everything we need to know about how to create and maintain a balanced blood pH level, and all the tips and tricks to make it easy and straightforward.

Are you ready to have a body operating at optimal health? Are you ready to get the most out of your diet? Are you ready to prevent disease and illness that you didn't even know you were susceptible to?

Then continue on reading on, because all of your questions are about to be answered.

Chapter 5: Creating an Acid-Alkaline Balance

In this chapter, we are going to take a look at some of the biggest and best ways to gain control of your acid-alkaline blood levels and ensure that you can maintain them at an optimal level. Many of the things that we are going to talk about here are not just about diet. In fact, even the alkaline diet is not just about diet — it is about habits. It is about keeping good habits, maintaining regular health goals, and being in tune with your own body.

There are plenty of signs and symptoms that you may notice in the event that your body is too acidic. It is very likely that you will be experiencing chronic fatigue if your body is too acidic. Even if it seems that though you have been sleeping enough, you may still feel this way. Other symptoms of overly acidic blood are pain, headaches, joint pain, and stiffness.

Generally, people with acidic blood express an overall feeling of sluggishness and lethargy — sometimes even depression. It is also associated with a sense of irritability and a dulling of the mental faculties.

Obviously, if you are experiencing any of these symptoms, it will be in your best interest to correct them to the best of your ability. There are lots of ways to make your blood more alkaline and we will look at a few here.

First of all, you will want to make sure that your symptoms or feelings are in fact coming from a pH imbalance. In order to do that, you will need to check your blood pH levels regularly in order to maintain an up-to-date record of your pH levels. You can do this very easily with simple, inexpensive home testing kits available online and at many drug stores. You can get an instant and highly accurate reading and find out exactly where your body's pH balance is sitting. These simple test kits can help you make healthy and informed decisions about your personal health based on accurate and current information. This is a great, convenient, and inexpensive way to always be on top of your health.

Now, before we get into specific diet plans, let us talk about some changes that we can make to our diet in a general sense that will help improve our blood pH levels. One such thing that we can do to ensure that we are maintaining appropriate levels of acidity in our blood is by making sure that we eat more greens and dark-colored vegetables in general. Greens are not always the most popular foods to eat despite their great reputation and association with good health. But there are ways to make greens and other veggies fun and exciting and taste great.

You could try new recipes and try new types of veggies that you have never tried before. If you already love veggies, try to make sure that you get a good amount on a regular basis, if not every day. Even if you have a particular proclivity for veggies, it's easy to leave them out on occasion. Try to avoid that tendency.

And if you don't like veggies, maybe it has something to do with a reduction in their appeal on account of processed foods and excessive artificial sugars. Simply by cutting these things out of our diets as much as possible can dramatically reduce cravings for said items and make good, nutrient-rich foods like dark, green veggies far more appealing.

Either way, try to experiment with new ways of getting your veggies and making them fun and enjoyable. Try keeping some prepared in advance so that you always have a quick and healthy snack.

Here is another quick tip for general health and well-being. Every morning, the first thing you do when you wake up should be to drink a great big glass of ice-cold water as fast as you can. Why? Well, it's quick and it's easy, it costs nothing, and it has all kinds of great health and wellness benefits both short-term and long-term. First of all, the most immediate benefit is that ice-cold blast of invigorating water will snap you wide awake quicker and more effectively than any caffeinated beverage.

What's more, there's nothing better than an icy surprise to jump-start your body and kick your metabolism into a high-gear first thing in the morning. And because our friend water is completely calorie-free, that basically amounts to an energy boost and metabolism enhancer for free, metabolically speaking.

And do you want to take this brilliant life hack one step further and bring it into our alkaline friendly lifestyle? Add just a touch of lemon to that morning burst of water, or better yet, all the water you drink and you will get all the previous benefits plus that boost to your body's alkalinity that you need to function at peak efficiency. This may seem counter-intuitive given that lemon is acidic, but remember, it is not always about the acid-alkaline balance of the compound itself. It is how our bodies metabolize that compound. And lemon, being a well-known metabolism booster, will give you that alkaline push you need.

Of course, sometimes it is about the actual acidity of the food we are eating. Specifically, it is about the amount of acidic foods we are eating. If you find that you are suffering from symptoms of acid reflux, kidney stones, low bone density, or anything else associated with high body acidity levels — that is almost certainly a strong indication that you should be strictly limiting your intake of acidic foods.

This goes of course for any of the obvious culprits like tomato sauce or spicy foods, but there are some less obvious foods that metabolize into an acidic by-product in our bodies that we should be cautious of as well. This includes many processed cakes and cereals, often grain such as rice, oats or pasta, and even certain nuts like peanuts or walnuts. The key here is to just always be aware of what we are consuming and keep everything in moderation.

Beverages as well should be kept in moderation especially coffee and alcohol since both of which are associated with many negative health effects when consumed in excess, far beyond body acid-alkaline balance.

Chapter 6: Alkaline Diet for Vegetarians

Don't let the title fool you, this isn't just for vegetarians. The alkaline diet is great for anyone and everyone. If you are already a vegetarian — great, you are already in a great spot to maintain an amazing alkaline diet. If you're not a vegetarian, that's okay too. Remember in the previous chapter when we said that it is not necessarily about how acidic the foods we eat are but the quantities? Well, that goes for meat. Most meats are extremely acid forming in our bodies.

That means that while they may not be acidic to the taste or even particularly acidic on a pH test, they metabolize in our bodies into an acidic by-product. So naturally, most alkaline diet meal plans are going to be either vegan or vegetarian, or just very light on the meat and dairy. That doesn't mean, of course, that you need to completely remove meat from your diet, but if you choose to continue eating meat, you will need to be highly aware of the quality and quantity of the meat you consume. Keep it moderate and make sure to maintain good health otherwise and you should be okay.

But speaking of acid-forming diets, what so bad about them? We have seen some of the symptoms of having a seriously acidic blood pH level, but what if we're just prone to eating a little bit on the acid-forming side? Well, simply by virtue of the fact that we live in a modern world with modern luxuries and modern conveniences, most of our diets have strayed away from a good, healthy acid-alkaline blood balance, and maybe some of us without even knowing it is may be living with a chronic condition that results from such a diet known as 'chronic low-grade metabolic acidosis'.

This is what happens when our diet leans to the slightly acidic side for an extended, if not an indefinite amount of time. And the reality is that unless we take active steps to counteract this condition, it is highly likely that we will all succumb to it eventually, if not already. That is just the nature of the world we live in and the habits and practices of the industries and populations of our societies.

So if you are suffering from a form of low-grade chronic metabolic acidosis, perhaps without even knowing it, what are the signs? For one thing, you may notice some weight gain. This is a result of inefficient metabolic function on account of long-term low-grade acidosis. You may also suffer from pronounced but unspecific aches and pains. These will often be in the joints or even the bones. This type of pain associated with low-grade acidosis is likely the result of an acid buildup in the joints and bones.

Acid reflux, predictably, is also a good sign of this prevalent condition. But that is not the only part of your digestive system that can be affected. Long-term, low-grade acidosis can also cause a number of other digestive issues like intestinal cramping, irritable bowel, and generally poor digestion.

A whole host of other issues could manifest if you are one of the high percentages of people who unknowingly live day to day with a chronic case of low-level metabolic acidosis. Chronic fatigue and a general feeling of tiredness and muscle weakness may result. As can a number of other issues like skin problems, bone loss, kidney stones, receding gums, and urinary tract problems. So if you find that you have three or more of the many possible symptoms, then at least eighty percent of your caloric intake should be from alkaline-forming foods. The remaining twenty percent can more or less be of your choosing, but you may find high protein food items to be helpful.

A nice, quick and easy way to boost your body's alkalinity is by drinking beverages that are alkalizing. Spring water is one such naturally occurring source of alkalizing water. Also, water with a dash of lemon juice just as mentioned earlier. Green tea or ginger root tea will also have a similarly alkalizing effect.

You'll want to make sure that you are focusing primarily on eating whole foods. So that means vegetables and fruits, as well as root crops like potatoes and turnips. Also nuts and seeds can be an excellent alkalizing source and also a very strong source of protein. Beans are generally a good choice as well, although lentils, in particular, are renowned for their excellent alkalize boost. And when consuming grains, just remember that it is always best to consume whole grains.

Whether you are pursuing an alkaline diet to target a specific issue, or if you just want to have the healthiest body you possibly can, you are going to want to eliminate as much processed and artificial foods as possible. In fact, that goes for everyone, no matter what. Processed and artificial foods are doing anybody any favors, but they will certainly cause your body's blood pH level to lean to the acidic side. Refined sugars and added sugars rank very high up on the list of these types of foods that should be avoided at all cost. And refined white flour isn't doing you any favors either. In fact, some say it can be just as bad as refined sugars.

And while we are on the topic of eliminating things, if you can handle giving up coffee or any other caffeinated beverages, you will be giving yourself a major advantage on the path to a balanced blood pH level.

There are certain foods and nutritional elements that are acid-forming but that our bodies still need to function properly. These are things that we will have to keep a particularly close eye on in order to monitor amounts of intake. This includes essential fats, as well as pasta and other grains. If you are choosing to continue eating meat, then it should also be noted that meat and fish should both be consumed very sparingly and should also be very closely monitored and limited.

Finally, when it comes to dressing up your greens, namely when being consumed as a salad or being cooked, make sure to use high-grade and healthy fats like extra-virgin, cold-pressed olive oil, avocado oil, and coconut oil. All of which bring along tons of health boosts and benefits in addition to their alkaline-forming properties.

Chapter 7: Alkaline Meal Ideas

Now that we are fully informed and equipped to make good nutrition choices in regard to acid-alkaline blood balance, it is now time to put together some meal plans so we can put all of what we have learned into practice. We are going to look at a prime example of everything you might eat in a day to get the most out of your body.

This particular example isn't about limiting calories of eliminating any particular foods or food groups, so if you have any particular calorie counts you need to stay within, or if you are eliminating certain food groups from your diet such as meat or dairy, you may have to adjust accordingly. Just make sure that if you're replacing anything, to replace it with something of a similar acid-alkaline value, and that it serves that same food role as the replaced item. That is to say, replace proteins with proteins, carbs with carbs, et cetera.

And if you are not calorie counting, obviously use your best judgment here but there is no limit to how many alkalizing foods in the fruits and vegetable categories you can eat. Certainly, you should be limiting acidic foods like meats, dairies, grains, and processed foods if for no reason than to keep your acidity levels down, but fruits and vegetables especially the ones that are particularly alkalizing, you can eat to your heart's content.

So with that said, let's take a look at what our alkaline diet morning might look like.

We wake up nice and early in the morning, refreshed and ready to tackle our day because our healthy, alkaline-rich diet is allowing us to get the sleep we need and preventing our bodies from feeling overly fatigued. The first thing we do is get an ice-cold glass of water, squeeze some fresh lemon juice into it and drink the whole thing as fast as we can. As fast as we can without getting a brain freeze that is!

So now we're going to want to have a nice satisfying breakfast. Today, we are going to do a veggie scramble. Sounds great, doesn't it? This breakfast is going to consist of one or two eggs that we are going to scramble up with green onions, spinach or bok choy or any other leafy greens, and then some chopped bell peppers and diced tomatoes. You can even try it as an omelet if you like. Or even an egg-white omelet if you're feeling really healthy.

Or better yet, if you really want to go healthy, why not try that same breakfast, but as a tofu scramble instead of scrambled eggs. It's easy and delicious. Just replace the eggs with a handful of diced, firm tofu. You can season your tofu however you like, but we recommend trying a chili-style seasoning for some nice, tex-mex style breakfast burritos. Wrap optional.

After that amazing breakfast, we're going to have a nice productive and active morning. If we feel the need for a snack before lunch, we'll have maybe a fruit like an apple or a pear, maybe a banana or a handful of nuts or seeds. An ideal choice would be pumpkin seeds or almonds.

If you're anything like us, that already sounds like an amazing and healthy, nutritious day, but we haven't even gotten to lunch yet. So what might we enjoy for our midday meal on this ideal alkaline diet day? Why limit ourselves, let's look at a couple of options.

For one, we could try some lentil soup. This packs a nice alkalizing punch as it is but combine that with some steamed green like broccoli, carrots, onions, or kale, and you've got a powerful meal. Heck, why not steam up a mix of all of those veggies. Try a light olive oil-based salad dressing on the steamed veggies for some extra flavor.

As delicious as that sounds though, we still have another option. If you're still of the animal eating persuasion, you could try a nice big salmon steak, still a far healthier choice that its terrestrial cousin, served with some mixed greens which could include cucumber, carrots, tomatoes, and broccoli, among pretty much any other fresh veggies you would like. Similarly, you can season that with a light vinaigrette of your choice, but we particularly recommend a lemon and dill based one.

After all that amazing nutrition, you must be ready for a snack! Fight off that mid-afternoon slump with a nice alkalizing snack. This one you can keep nice and simple. Try a simple hard-boiled egg, seasoned with sea salt and fresh ground pepper to taste and a garnish of your choice if you're feeling fancy. Or if you're not inclined toward the animal-based foods, try a straightforward but delicious snack consisting of strips of sweet bell peppers, celery, or carrots, or a mix of all is always an option!

Finally, it's time for dinner and this is where you remaining meat eaters are going to have your way. You can have up to four ounces of your favorite meat, whatever that might be, but we highly recommend that if you must have meat, try to stick to something along the lines of fish, chicken, or other types of light poultry. You can serve this with a side of yam or sweet potatoes, baked or prepared in your favorite way and a nice simple garden salad with mixed greens and a light dressing of your choice.

Or for the plant-based folks, you can indulge in some pasta, but try to find or make pasta made from rice or quinoa, or other grains than wheat. Then you can top your pasta with all kinds of delicious veggies like broccoli, zucchini, and garlic. And then garnish with some olive oil and salt and pepper. Now you've had yourself a fresh and healthy food day!

CONCLUSION

Thanks for making it all of the way through to the very end of *Thyroid Healing: The Proven 4 Week Program to Improve Your Metabolism, Hypothyroidism, Hormones, Tiredness, and Weight Gain*. It is my sincere hope as the author, that reading through all of this was informative for you, and that you perhaps even got a little more than you bargained for on your journey, and now feel well equipped to tackle whatever lies ahead for you.

For this is not truly the end is it, but merely a small step in a forward direction. It is now time to utilize what you have learned going through these pages, and all that the knowledge contained within has to offer. If you or a loved one you know has, has had, or may seem to have a thyroid issue, every tool that is needed to aid them or yourself in the journey forward is now at your fingertips.

Now is when it is time to go see a doctor, to make sure that information is properly communicated. It is never too late, and never a bad idea, especially where the thyroid gland is concerned, to set oneself up with a regular and balanced diet, as well as having a plan for daily exercise in a range of activities.

The next step is to put everything that you have learned in this book into practice. Learning more about your body and how it works is always a great place to start and in this book, we learned all about the acid-alkaline balance in our bodies, how the chemistry works, and what are the effects this balance or imbalance can have on our health.

We learned about some of the cutting edge science behind our understanding of pH levels in our body, and how we can fine tune them to the perfect level through our diet and other important practices. The human body is a very complicated and delicate machine, but the more we come to understand it, the better off we are and the more educated we can be in our choices regarding our health and wellbeing.